THE ARTHRITIS DIET

Anti-Inflammatory Foods That Relieve Arthritis and Reduce Joint Inflammation

Table of Contents

Introduction

We want to thank you for purchasing the book, "The Arthritis Diet: Anti-Inflammatory Foods That Relieve Arthritis and Joint Inflammation". Congratulations on taking the first step toward improving your health.

This book discusses various foods that can help you overcome the pain of arthritis and deal with general inflammation. It includes information designed to help you make an informed decision as you work toward implementing an "arthritis diet". We have provided a comprehensive list of foods that will help to reduce inflammation in your body, as well as some foods that are known to cause inflammation and should possibly be avoided. The foods discussed here are grouped according to their type (fruits/vegetables, oils, etc.), and each food section explains not only how a particular item manages arthritis and/or reduces inflammation, but also what the health benefits are and how you can incorporate that particular food or food group into your diet, with the goal being to help you design a diet plan that will reduce inflammation and help you to feel better. We are confident that once you are finished with this book you'll be on your way to creating an "arthritis diet" that will significantly reduce your pain and improve your quality of life.

Thank you again for downloading this book. We hope that you find it informative and helpful as you make decisions related to your food choices. As with any diet plan, please make sure you discuss your concerns and choices with your physician, to ensure that you are making the best possible decisions for your health issues.

Chapter 1: About the Arthritis Diet

What an Arthritis Diet Should Do for You

Although the focus of this book is on foods that can address arthritis and joint inflammation, it would do you well to know what to look for when considering whether or not to include a particular food or food group in your diet. Ultimately, your aim is to have an "Arthritis diet" that helps you to focus on your whole body, rather than just one specific area. Ideally, your food choices should be able to:

<u>Help Curb Inflammation</u>

Arthritis is characterized by inflammation, which is the body's attempt to protect itself. Harmful stimuli, including an injury, pathogen, damaged cells or irritants can all cause inflammation. Acute inflammation is an indication that the body is trying to heal itself. Eating foods that relieve the inflammation in your body will help expedite the healing process. It is important to note that the presence of inflammation does not automatically mean that there is an infection in the body. Infection is caused by bacteria, a virus or fungus, and inflammation is simply and indication that the body is aware of the problem and is trying to fight it.

Inflammation is not always bad, and it is important to distinguish between the two types of inflammation that may be present in the body.

- Acute inflammation comes on suddenly, and is the result of an illness or injury to the body. It may be present for a few hours, days or weeks, however it is usually not a permanent condition.

- Chronic inflammation is a long-term condition that can result from not treating acute inflammation, as an autoimmune response to otherwise healthy tissue, or as the result of an irritant that persists over a period of time.

Protect Against Autoimmune Diseases

Autoimmune diseases such as Lupus, Fibromyalgia, Celiac Disease, Graves Disease and literally hundreds of others are caused when the body initiates an immune response to healthy cells. Inflammation occurs as the body attempts to fight the "imagined" threat to its systems. Acute inflammation is nearly always a part of an autoimmune disease, and some researchers believe that acute and prolonged inflammation in the body can actually trigger an autoimmune disease.

Help You Manage or Lose Weight and Reduce the Strain on Your Joints.

If you are struggling to lose weight, recent studies indicate that there may be inflammation running unchecked in your body. A diet high in processed foods, which contain high amounts of sugar and fats, can lead to inflammation and cause your weight to balloon. This excess weight places a strain on your joints, which then initiate an immune response to fix the problem.

Recognizing your unhealthy eating patterns and initiating changes in your diet can help to decrease the inflammation in your body, leading to a gradual weight loss and reducing the strain on your joints. Prolonged stress and strain on your joints can lead you to develop arthritis, turning a temporary condition into a permanent one.

Substances That Relieve Arthritis and Reduce Inflammation

There are many compounds in food that are believed to have anti-inflammatory properties. Here are some of the more common ones, as well as the foods in which they are found.

Omega-3 Fatty Acids

Also known as PUFAs or polyunsaturated fatty acids, omega-3s are essential fatty acids. They are necessary for a healthy body, however the body cannot produce them naturally and so they must be obtained from food sources. Omega-3s can be found in healthy oils (e.g. olive oil, grapeseed oil, and safflower oil), fish oils, and fatty/oily fish (e.g. salmon, albacore tuna, sardines, and herring).

Omega-3 fatty acids first became popular because they help keep the heart healthy. Recent studies have shown that they may be able to reduce inflammation and alleviate symptoms of rheumatoid arthritis and osteoarthritis.

Vitamins that Fight Inflammation

Antioxidant vitamins such as C, D and E have properties that have been shown to fight inflammation in the body and reduce the harmful effects of free radicals.

Vitamin A – Found in vegetables such as kale, sweet potatoes, spinach, carrots, broccoli and collard greens, as well as in beef liver, and milk, this vitamin has been shown to effectively reduce inflammation in the body when paired with beta-carotene, a provitamin that converts to Vitamin A in the body.

Vitamin C – Studies have shown that increased or adequate vitamin C intake reduces the level of C-reactive proteins or CRP in the blood. CRP is a marker for inflammation that is present when there are high levels of inflammation present in the body.

Vitamin E – This vitamin is found in green leafy vegetables, sunflower seeds, almonds and avocados, and can also be taken as a supplement. Some experts believe that vitamin E causes inflammatory substances that cause damage to the heart to be released more slowly into the body, minimizing the effect that they have on the system and reducing the risk of cardiovascular disease. The alpha-tocopherol form of vitamin E has also been found to reduce lung inflammation in animals.

Quercetin

Found in onions, tea, citrus fruits, and apples, quercetin is a flavonoid that contains antioxidant properties. It eases inflammation by inhibiting inflammatory agents, including histamines, leukotrienes, and prostaglandins, which are substances in the body that cause inflammation and can lead to conditions such as osteoarthritis and autoimmune diseases like rheumatoid arthritis and lupus.

Anthocyanin

Like quercetin, anthocyanin is also a flavonoid with antioxidant properties. This plant pigment is found in purple and red fruits, including blueberries, raspberries, and cherries. Anthocyanins are believed to have antioxidant and more importantly, anti-inflammatory properties. They prevent inflammation by neutralizing enzymes and inhibiting oxidants that cause damage to the blood vessels' connective tissues. When these tissues are destroyed, blood leaks into other tissues, causing pain and inflammation. They also ease inflammation by repairing damaged blood vessels and thereby putting a stop to blood leakage.

There are food sources containing the substances above that are not discussed in this book. The inclusion of this chapter is meant to guide you towards choosing foods that will provide you with the right nutrients to address arthritis and/or reduce joint inflammation, however we strongly recommend that you do diligent research to ensure that you are choosing the proper foods for your body.

Foods That May Worsen Inflammation

Foods High in Trans Fat

Processed food and junk food contain trans fats. These are man made fats that are used in processed foods to increase shelf life, and decrease refrigeration requirements. Trans fats are produced through "partial hydrogenation" or the addition of hydrogen atoms to unsaturated fats. This results in partially hydrogenated fat or trans fat which can be used repeatedly, and which lasts longer and is less expensive than the non-hydrogenated variety. These qualities made trans fat the go-to fat of many food manufacturers – never mind its negative impact on health.

Trans fat increases the risk of heart disease and raises LDL or "bad" cholesterol levels in the body. It also causes the immune system to be overactive, resulting in unwanted inflammation that is has been implicated in any number of conditions including diabetes, cardiovascular disease and strokes.

Food High in Saturated Fat

Saturated fat occurs naturally in nature. The most well known sources are red meat, and full-fat dairy products. Beef, cheese, ice cream, butter, and pizza all contain saturated fats, and while your body needs fats to run properly, you must be very careful to monitor the amount of fat in your diet. Saturated fat is considered to be the "bad" fat. It raises cholesterol levels in the blood, which in turn increases your risk of developing heart disease. It may also lead to weight gain because foods rich in it are usually high in calories.

Research on dietary factors that either promoted or hindered inflammation has shown that there is a direct correlation between intake of saturated fat and inflammation and C-reactive protein (CRP) levels. A diet that is primarily made up of foods that contain saturated fats, as well as a diet high in processed foods, increases your risk of inflammation in the body, potentially leading to the development of autoimmune disease, diabetes, cardiovascular disease and osteoarthritis, just to name a few.

Nightshade Vegetables

The nightshade family includes bell peppers, eggplants, (white) potatoes, and tomatoes. The link between consuming nightshade veggies and inflammation is still weak, and for this reason some experts advise against eliminating nightshade vegetables from your diet altogether because you will potentially miss out on their nutritional benefits. In some studies, subjects suffering from inflammation reported that avoiding the said food items had a positive effect. If you seek relief from arthritis or joint inflammation try abstaining from nightshade vegetables for a period of time and see if doing so yields a positive result.

Chapter 2: Fruits and Vegetables That Relieve Arthritis and Reduce Inflammation

Apples

"An apple a day keeps the doctor away". Turns out that our grandmothers may have been on to something. Apples have the second highest levels of antioxidants of any known fruit, and are rich in phytochemicals, which help to reduce inflammation in the body. They are also an important source of boron, an important trace element that has been proven instrumental in the fight against osteoarthritis.

Health Benefits

Apples are nutrient powerhouses. They are a good source of vitamins A and C, which promote eye health and improve your resistance against diseases. They are also replete with antioxidants, which prevent free radicals from wreaking havoc on your cells and causing health conditions ranging from heart disease to cancer.

Apples also contain pectin, a dietary fiber that comes together when it's in the intestinal tract. This makes you feel fuller, and thus may curb food cravings - making these fruits a wise choice for those looking to lose weight.

How Apples Help to Ease Inflammation

In a recent study, participants were instructed to add ¾ cup of dried apples to their daily diet for one year. The results showed that they reduced their "bad" cholesterol (LDL) levels by almost 23% while registering an improvement of between 3 and 5% in their "good" cholesterol (HDL). Participants also displayed lower C-reactive protein or CRP levels in their blood, reducing their levels of inflammation in the body.

CRP is a key marker for inflammation. When you have a high amount of this protein in your blood, a part of your body is inflamed. Studies also found that CRP has a direct hand in worsening inflammation in conditions such as atherosclerosis.

Adding More Apples to Your Diet

Apples are a delicious and healthier alternative to the usual high-calorie and high-fat snacks. You can eat them as is, or slice/chop them up and add to salads and even sandwiches. There are also a lot of desserts that make use of them.

As much as possible leave the peel on apples; otherwise you won't get their full antioxidant benefits. Also, choose apples that are still firm and crunchy – over-ripeness causes the pectin in them to break down and makes them mushy. Apples are also on the "dirty dozen" list—those fruits and vegetables known to be high in pesticides—so be sure to buy organic when at all possible, or wash your produce well.

Cherries

Native to the regions of Asia Minor and Eastern Europe, cherries (particularly tart or Montmorency cherries) or "drupes" (i.e., stone fruits) are known for their ability to reduce pain and inflammation as well as boost recovery time in patients with injuries that have caused inflammation in the body. Cherries are also high in antioxidants, and are among the few foods known to contain the potent anti-cancer phytochemical perillyl alcohol.

Health Benefits

Cherries are rich in vitamins A and C that boost the immune system and improve eyesight, among other things. They also contain potassium that not only lowers blood pressure, but also promotes overall health by improving the function of several organs including the brain, heart, and kidneys. Cherries likewise have melatonin, a naturally occurring hormone that triggers the anticipation of darkness in the body and helps regulate sleep cycles.

How Cherries Relieve Arthritis and Inflammation

There is still much research to be done to determine exactly how cherries fight inflammation, but recent studies are showing a lot of promise. Research has shown that cherries – whether eaten fresh or ingested as pills – address inflammation in two ways. First, by preventing recurrent attacks – which include inflammation as a symptom - in people with gout by reducing uric acid in the blood. And second, consumption of cherries results in decreased CRP levels – and therefore, decreased inflammation - in people suffering from osteoarthritis. Experts believe that both of these results are due to the anthocyanins in cherries.

<u>Adding Cherries to Your Diet</u>

Cherries can be found in many forms, and all of these provide the same benefits of increasing anthocyanins and lowering CRP levels in the body. You can snack on a handful of fresh cherries every day, or include these in your smoothies. You can also bake with them. Cherry juice is an excellent source of their benefits; however make sure that you choose an all-natural juice and not one that is loaded with sugar. Health food stores carry a liquid extract, which can be used in cooking or added to drinks, as well as cherry pills, which can be taken daily to manage inflammation.

Pineapples

Pineapples are rich in the enzyme bromelain, which has been proven to have a powerful affect on pain, as well as reducing swelling and inflammation in the body. Pineapples can be eaten fresh, canned or frozen, however it is important to note that most canned pineapple has added sugar.

Strawberries

Strawberries are a mainstay in many people's grocery list. They are a popular component in various desserts and sweet dishes, and are a delicious and healthy snack. These fruits should be included in your "arthritis diet" not only because of their anti-inflammatory properties but also because of their numerous health benefits.

Health Benefits

Strawberries reduce your risk of stroke and heart disease by reducing the amount of C-reactive protein or CRP in your blood. One study found that people with high CRP levels are more prone to developing inflammation related conditions and those who increased their consumption of strawberries had a lower amount of CRP in their body.

How Strawberries Relieve Arthritis

Strawberries ease arthritis symptoms – in particular, inflammation – by lowering the CRP levels in the blood. The presence of CRP in high amounts indicates inflammation; when this protein is reduced, inflammation is abated.

Adding Strawberries to Your Diet

It is not at all difficult to add strawberries to your list of food staples. You can eat them as is, or add them to salads and smoothies. You can use them as toppings for your morning cereal/oatmeal, too. If you want to try something new you can also add strawberries to your vinaigrettes. Strawberries are part of the "dirty dozen" list—those fruits and vegetables highest in pesticide residue, so be sure to buy organic when possible.

Papaya

Christopher Columbus called papaya "the fruit of the angels". These vitamin and mineral powerhouses also contain a substance called papain, which has been shown in numerous studies to be as effective, if not more so, than many over-the-counter medications in reducing inflammation and pain. Throw papaya in your juicer with an apple, a carrot and a banana for a nutrient rich smoothie to get your day started off right.

Onions

Onions are found almost everything we eat. They are low in calories and are virtually fat-free. Whether or not you are suffering from inflammation, these vegetables are worth a space in your pantry.

Health Benefits

Onions are rich in flavonoids--antioxidants that prevent cell damage caused by free radicals, which is why experts believe they may have anti-cancer properties. They are also good for the heart as they can reduce the levels of bad cholesterol (i.e., low-density lipoprotein or LDL cholesterol) in the body. Finally, onions may prevent bone loss, too, due to a compound found in them known as GPCS.

How Onions Fight Inflammation

The quercetin in onions is responsible for the vegetables' anti-inflammatory properties. As mentioned in the first part of this book, this compound inhibits the substances that cause inflammation in chronic conditions such as rheumatoid arthritis and osteoarthritis.

How to Incorporate More Onions in Your Diet

There are a lot of dishes that call for the addition of onions, so incorporating these vegetables in your diet isn't hard to do. The only thing left to consider is the kind you should use.

Unless a dish specifically calls for sweet or white onions, go for varieties with a strong flavor and smell. This is because shallots, as well as red and yellow onions, were found to have higher levels of beneficial compounds compared to other, more subtle varieties.

Chapter 3: Protein Sources, Nuts and Grains That Address Arthritis and Inflammation

Fatty Fish

Fatty or oily fish are cold-water fish. They differ from white fish in that their whole body contains oil, while the latter only have oil in their liver. They should be a staple in any "arthritis diet" because they contain nutrients that effectively deal with inflammation and diseases such as arthritis. Examples of fatty fish are the following: eel, herring, kipper, mackerel, salmon, sardines, trout, and tuna.

Health Benefits

Consumption of fatty or oily fish will provide you with high amounts of omega-3 fatty acids and lean protein. Fatty fish lower triglyceride levels in your body. It reduces your risk of developing chronic conditions (such as heart disease and rheumatoid arthritis) as well as certain types of cancer (most specifically, oral and skin cancers). It helps improve your memory, and it can also protect you against vision loss and even dementia later in life.

How Fatty Fish Reduce Inflammation

Fatty fish are an excellent source of omega-3s or polyunsaturated fatty acids (PUFAs), which, as mentioned in the first chapter of this book, not only ease inflammation but also reduce symptoms of arthritis. Omega-3s do this by promoting the production of resolvins - a type of fat that may prevent inflammation.

Tips for Consuming Fatty Fish

Buy wild caught rather than farmed fish. Fish that are raised on farms are fed a diet of grains (mostly corn) that is unhealthy for them as well as for you. Look for fish that say, "wild caught" on the packaging to ensure that your fish grew up eating the foods that nature intended.

Prepare them properly. Deep-frying fatty fish is not recommended as this can strip them of some of their nutrients. For optimum health benefits, fish should be steamed, baked or grilled. Frying fish is unhealthy, as it raises the fat content of the dish and potentially adds trans fats to your food.

Choose wisely. Although fresh fish is preferable, you can use canned or frozen fatty fish and still enjoy their many health benefits. If you find a good source of fresh fish, make sure you pick those that smell of the sea, have clear, bright eyes, and flesh that is firm to the touch.

Eat in moderation. Constantly going over the recommended 8 ounces of fatty fish per week can lead to weight gain; after all, oily fish are obviously high in fats. It may also put you in danger, as there are some fatty fish varieties that contain toxic substances such as mercury and PCBs or polychlorinated biphenyls. Again, ensure that you are choosing the healthiest options by purchasing the freshest fish possible, and only eating those varieties that say "wild caught" on the label.

Walnuts

Walnuts have the highest concentration of Omega-3 fatty acids of any nut on the planet. They have also been shown to inhibit the production of neurotransmitters, which can increase inflammation and cause pain in the body.

Health Benefits

Walnuts are rich in fiber, unsaturated fat, protein, vitamin E, and antioxidants. They also supply the body with copper and manganese. Unlike other nuts, walnuts contain high amounts of omega-3 fatty acids.

Walnuts do a lot for the body. They promote heart and bone health, and improve blood flow to your muscles. They also prevent cell damage caused by free radicals. Walnuts are likewise believed to have anti-cancer properties.

How Walnuts Relieve Arthritis and Ease Inflammation

Omega-3 fatty acids in animal products – specifically in fish oils – are known to reduce joint pain and inflammation in rheumatoid arthritis. It is still unclear whether the omega-3s in walnuts produce similar results, but in a related study it was found that people who increase their intake of these nuts are able to reduce the levels of C-reactive protein (CRP) in their blood. This means that walnuts may be able to ease inflammation, too.

Incorporating Walnuts into Your Diet

Most people consume walnuts by using them in desserts and snacking on them as is. But there are other ways by which you can include them in your diet. You can add them to your morning oats or cereal, or to your daily dose of yogurt. They also add flavor and crunch to ice cream. And they need not be confined to sweet fare. They can be chopped and included in salads, cooked rice, couscous, and even sautéed vegetables. You can likewise create a walnut-based dip for vegetable sticks and nachos.

Whole Grains

Whole and refined grains are similar in that they are both cereal grains. The difference lies in their composition. Refined grains such as white flour and white bread only make use of the cereal grain's endosperm – that is, the protective covering of the germ or the plant embryo. Whole grains, on the other hand, include all the parts of the grain, namely: the endosperm, the germ, and the outer layer or the bran. Examples of whole grains are brown rice, quinoa, and oats. They also include wholegrain products like whole wheat bread and flour.

Health Benefits

Whole grains are high in dietary fiber – making them a very effective weight loss tool. They also provide magnesium, iron, selenium, and several B vitamins.

Consuming whole grains has a positive effect on your overall health. These foods keep your brain and heart healthy. They also boost your immune system, and reduce your risk of developing chronic conditions.

How Whole Grains Provide Relief from Arthritis

The positive effect of whole grain consumption on inflammation is well documented. A study done in Germany established that people who do not consume a lot of whole grains during pre-adolescence are prone to having higher levels of interleukin-6 (which indicates the presence of inflammation in the body) during adulthood. Related studies showed similar results: intake of whole grain products has a direct correlation to the levels of inflammation markers such as C-reactive proteins or CRP in the blood. Simply put, when you eat more whole grains, your CRP levels decrease, which means inflammation is reduced. In another study, this time done in the US, it was found that consumption of whole grains led to a decrease in systemic inflammation.

A Tip on Incorporating Whole Grains into Your Diet

If you're not used to eating whole grain products you might find it hard to incorporate them into your diet because of their texture. To make the transition easier, replace refined grains with whole grain products gradually.

Chapter 4: Healthy Oils That Fight Inflammation

Liquid oils, such as the ones discussed below, are better for your heart and your health in general compared to solid fats like butter and margarine. Quite a number of them can also help you fight inflammation, which may either be a precursor to several chronic diseases or brought about by a condition such as arthritis.

Avocado Oil

Green and mild tasting, this healthy oil derived from the avocado fruit has yet to become a kitchen staple in many households. Given its many benefits, though, you might want to give this healthy oil a try.

<u>Health Benefits</u>

Avocado is a high fat fruit...but it's a good fat. One avocado contains almost 22 grams of monounsaturated fat and provides an excellent nutrition boost for any meal that it is added to. Avocados also boost the absorption of various nutrients found in other food because of its high unsaturated fat content, as well as raise the levels of HDL or good cholesterol and lower blood pressure in the body.

Avocado oil is likewise being looked into as a natural cure for psoriasis and periodontal disease.

How It Helps

This healthy oil reduces inflammation by reducing the levels of C-reactive protein (CRP) in the blood. Research that was done in Europe indicated that a supplement that combined soybean oil and avocado oil extracts successfully improved arthritis and osteoarthritis symptoms. So convincing are the results of this study that the said supplement is now recognized as a prescription drug in France.

How to Use Avocado Oil

Avocado oil has a mild flavor, and it is easy to find ways to incorporate it into your diet. Use it instead of olive oil for your pesto sauce and other pesto-based dishes. You can also use it as a bread dip, and it makes for a great base in vinaigrettes. And since avocado oil has a high smoke point, it can likewise be used for stir-frying. There are many "flavored" avocado oils available in the gourmet section of your grocery store, and these make an excellent cooking substitution for other "less healthy" oils.

Grapeseed Oil

Grapeseed oil is a by-product of the winemaking process. Also known as grape oil, it is produce by pressing the grape seeds – in particular, the ones that have been discarded during winemaking. It is usually extracted chemically since each grape seed yields only a very small amount of oil. Grapeseed oil is known for its culinary and cosmetic uses.

Health Benefits

Grapeseed oil contains an omega-9 fatty acid called oleic acid that has been shown to help control food cravings. This makes it an effective tool for losing and managing weight. It was also found to reduce bad cholesterol or LDL levels and raise good cholesterol levels in the body.

How It Helps

Grapeseed oil is an excellent source of polyunsaturated fats or omega-3 fatty acids and vitamin E – substances known to have anti-inflammatory properties.

How to Use Grapeseed Oil

Grapeseed oil is perfect for cooking – even high-heat cooking - due to its high smoke point. It also has a light, clean taste that makes it ideal for marinades for fish, poultry, and other meats.

Olive Oil

Olive oil is undoubtedly the best-known healthy oil in this chapter. It is a staple in different cuisines around the world, and brings added flavor to many dishes. It also provides a host of health benefits that should convince you to give this oil a permanent place in your pantry.

Health Benefits

Olive oil has many health benefits. It contains polyphenolic compounds, which promote heart health, and hydroxytyrosol, which was found to protect the nervous system against diseases. Recently it was established that when mixed with vitamin D, olive oil could help to prevent bone loss.

How It Relieves Inflammation

Olive oil contains oleocanthal, a substance that is believed to have the same effect as NSAIDs or non-steroidal anti-inflammatory drugs such as aspirin and ibuprofen. Oleocanthal works the same way as ibuprofen by blocking the production of COX-1 and COX-2 – enzymes that promote inflammation and increase the body's pain sensitivity.

Incorporating Olive Oil Into Your Diet

Choose wisely. The effectiveness of olive oil in reducing pain and inflammation is directly related to its "throaty bite" – that is, the peppery, ticklish feeling it provides at the back of the throat when it is ingested. If you want to enjoy its full benefits, choose cold pressed, extra virgin olive oil.

Use it properly. Olive oil is not meant to be used in high-heat cooking (such as stir-frying) since this will reduce its healthy qualities. You may use it for sautéing and frying, though. Room temperature olive oil can be used as a bread dip, in salad dressings, and for tossing pasta.

Consume in moderation. If you plan on substituting ibuprofen with olive oil, make sure you modify your diet to accommodate the extra calories you'll be ingesting. A 200-milligram ibuprofen tablet is equivalent to 3.5 tablespoons of olive oil, which is a whopping 400 calories or more. Stay away from fatty food while you're taking this healthy oil as medication.

Safflower Oil

Safflower oil is derived from the seeds of the safflower plant. It has two variants: high-linoleic and high oleic. The former is best used in unheated food since it contains polyunsaturated fats/omega-3s. The latter, on the other hand, is rich in monounsaturated fats and can be used in place of olive oil in cooking.

Health Benefits

Safflower oil is high in vitamin E, which has antioxidant properties, and polyunsaturated fats/omega-3 fatty acids. Experts believe that both of these substances provide a number of health benefits, including lowering cholesterol and blood sugar levels in the body. They may also reduce abdominal fat, which makes safflower oil effective in weight loss and management.

How It Eases Inflammation

Like the other healthy oils in this chapter, safflower oil is said to have anti-inflammatory qualities because of the omega-3 fatty acids and vitamin E it contains.

How to Use Safflower Oil

It is recommended that you consume at least 1 2/3 teaspoon of safflower oil daily to enjoy its many benefits. Considering it has a neutral taste, this isn't hard to do at all. You can use it to make salad dressings, as well as oil-based spreads and dips. An easy and delicious way to incorporate safflower oil into your diet is to blend it with lemon juice and fresh basil. Then, drizzle the mixture over baked, pan-friend, and even steamed fish.

Coconut oil

Coconut oil has been in the news lately for it's seemingly endless health and wellness abilities. Long thought unhealthy because of its high fat content, coconut oil is now known to be high in antioxidants, with some studies showing them to be more effective than non-steroidal pain medication at relieving pain and inflammation in the body.

Coconut oil has a high smoke point, making it an excellent choice for cooking. Be sure to choose virgin coconut oil, as refined oils have had most of their healing properties stripped away during the refinement process.

Chapter 5: Other Foods That Relieve Arthritis and Reduce Inflammation

Turmeric

Turmeric is primarily used as an essential ingredient in curries. Aside from serving as a spice in many dishes, it is also used as a pigment and as medicine for various health conditions.

Health Benefits

Turmeric is rich in manganese and iron. It can also provide you with dietary fiber, potassium, and vitamin B6. Studies suggest that it may have anti-cancer properties. It can also protect against several skin conditions, stomach ulcers, diabetes, and even Alzheimer's disease. It is likewise used in alternative medicine to treat depression.

How It Helps Fight Inflammation

Turmeric contains polyphenolic compounds called curcuminoids, which are responsible for its yellow hue. Curcumin is the primary curcuminoid and the most active substance in turmeric. It is also the focus of many studies on the health benefits – in particular, the anti-inflammatory properties – of the said rhizome.

Research has established that curcumin combats inflammation at a molecular level. It blocks the protein complex NF-KB, which plays a hand in the immune system's response to infection. When incorrectly regulated, this protein is known to cause inflammation and more serious conditions such as autoimmune diseases and cancer. Simply put, turmeric consumption prevents inflammation by blocking its source.

How to Add Turmeric to Your Diet

Aside from cooking curries with it, turmeric can also be used sparingly to add color and flavor in rice dishes, egg salads, soups, and sauces. There is also turmeric tea, which you can drink after meals for a nutrition boost.

Capsicum/Cayenne Pepper

Cayenne pepper has a long history of use both as a medicine and as a cooking ingredient. Native Americans have been using these spices for thousands of years, while Asian healers have known of its curative properties for centuries.

Health Benefits

Cayenne pepper is high in capsaicin, and contains the following nutrients: vitamin B6, vitamin C, vitamin E, manganese, and potassium. These and other capsicums are a proven digestive aid. They are also used to address various conditions affecting the blood vessels and the heart: they lower cholesterol levels, improve blood circulation, and even prevent the onset of cardiovascular disease.

Capsicum is sometimes applied to the skin to reduce muscle spasms and nerve pain. It's also used to lessen pain resulting from rheumatoid arthritis, shingles, and fibromyalgia.

How Cayenne Pepper Helps Reduce Inflammation

Cayenne pepper and other capsicums contain capsaicin. A study of this compound and its effects has shown that it can provide relief from pain and inflammation in individuals suffering from arthritis and osteoarthritis. Cayenne pepper also contains the antioxidants carotenoids and flavonoids. These neutralize free radicals, which induce inflammation by damaging/destroying the cells in the body.

Tips for Consuming Cayenne Pepper

Store it properly. Dried and ground peppers should be stored in airtight containers and kept in a cool, dark place.

Handle it with care. The capsaicin in cayenne pepper can cause pain if it enters the eye. It may also trigger a burning sensation on the spot of skin where it's applied, so it is important that you handle capsicums with care. Wear gloves and/or goggles if you'll be dealing with a lot of peppers, and wash your hands after handling them to prevent accidents.

Consider the fact that it is a nightshade vegetable. In the beginning of this book it was mentioned that some people avoid nightshade vegetables because of the belief that they exacerbate inflammation. If eliminating these veggies had a positive effect on your health, it might be best to not include cayenne peppers and other capsicums in your "arthritis diet".

Tea

More and more people are switching to tea instead of coffee because it is thought to be healthier. It contains less caffeine, and provides numerous health benefits. It may also address inflammation, so it should definitely be added to your arthritis diet.

Health Benefits

Tea promotes bone and hearth health. It also has antioxidant and anti-inflammatory properties. It is no surprise, then, that it should be included in your arthritis diet. There are different kinds of tea, but all of these contain antioxidants that protect the body from free radicals. Tea is likewise calorie-free, so those suffering from inflammation brought about by diseases such as rheumatoid arthritis and osteoarthritis can enjoy its benefits without gaining weight. In some cases drinking tea, especially green tea, may also help in weight loss because it is know to boost your metabolism. These are noteworthy benefits because as mentioned earlier, being overweight or obese exacerbates inflammation and may even increase the odds of developing arthritis and other chronic conditions.

How Tea Eases Inflammation

White Tea. A study of various teas and their effects found that white tea is the healthiest and contains the most polyphenols - probably because it is not as processed as oolong and black tea. It provides relief from inflammation by inhibiting elastase and collagenase – enzymes that encourage inflammation by damaging connective tissues.

Green Tea. Green tea contains about the same amount of polyphenols as white tea. It is rich in EGCG or epigallocatechin gallate – a polyphenol that has been found to successfully halt the progression of arthritis by preventing interleukin-1 from breaking down cartilage. Interleukin-1 is a blood cell that supposedly helps the body fight infections by producing inflammation.

Tea Consumption Tips

Brew tea the right way. To get the most out of drinking tea, make sure you brew it properly by steeping a tea bag or tea leaves in water (boiled, not boiling) for about 5 minutes. You can drink it hot or iced, plain or with honey and lemon – it will still give you the same benefits.

Complement it with other healthy food. Polyphenols give tea most of its benefits. However, studies showed that the polyphenol levels in your blood will drop a mere two hours after taking your last sip. To keep this from happening you'd have to drink about 8 cups of tea over the course of a day, which is very hard to do. You'd need to add other sources in your diet to maintain elevated polyphenol levels in your body.

You have many choices. White and green teas may have the highest amount of polyphenols, but other kinds can still provide you with the same benefits. What matters here is you make tea a part of your arthritis diet.

Conclusion

We hope that you have found this book to be beneficial as you set out to reduce the inflammation in your body and begin to heal! Remember...this is all a process. It's a marathon, not a sprint. Begin making small changes in your diet and lifestyle, and work your way up to a more healthy and balanced way of living. Incorporating even one change a week can help you change your habits and make new ones, and in just a short time you'll be feeling better...both physically and emotionally.

The next step you need to take is to create an "arthritis diet" for yourself based on the facts presented to you in this book, and the research that you have conducted on your own. We have provided suggestions here for foods that can be incorporated into your diet to help heal your inflammation and arthritis pain, however the real task is up to you. Consider your likes and dislikes, and talk with your primary care physician or nutritionist to help create an eating plan that will get you back on the road to good health. When your diet is made up of your own choices, rather than dictated by someone else, you have a better chance of meeting your goals.

Changing how and what you eat is not easy, so don't feel angry or frustrated if you find yourself succumbing to your old habits in the beginning. Whenever you feel like sticking to your new diet plan is an impossible task, recall the reasons for your decision to eat healthy, and picture yourself feeling better and enjoying life to it's fullest. Remember...there is no substitute for living a full, healthy life centered on being with your loved ones and enjoying the beautiful planet that we live on. By changing your diet, you are taking the first step toward a new, more fulfilling life...one in which you feel better about yourself and your choices.

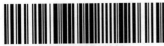

Made in the USA
Middletown, DE
30 May 2019